The Eatsy Way to Live

Lose Weight, Change Your Life

By: Thomas Warren

Introduction & Disclaimer: I wrote this book to help people. I had a problem that 1/3 Americans are currently facing: I was obese. I found a solution and I am presenting my solution. I am not a doctor or nutrition expert. Thank you to my family, girlfriend and friends for support. Good luck.

Chapter 1

I have spoken with many doctors about weight loss, along with personal trainers. I have collected the essentials for losing weight that is why I created this diet. I want to share my collection of knowledge with anyone who needs help. This diet will teach you about what is going in to your body, along with some easy tricks to help speed up the weight loss process.

At one point a doctor told me that if I did not lose 50lbs that I was at serious risk of diabetes and other health problems. It was at that moment almost 10 years ago that I started to try every weight loss solution available to me.

If you are a horrible eater then be prepared to have the easiest time with this diet and see the quickest results. If you already eat decently, then the second chapter will be the key to your weight lost.

This guide will show you how to lose weight relatively quickly by changing your diet, unconventionally, and introducing a new form of exercise that is directed towards weight loss (as opposed to muscle gain).

It is important that you follow the first three chapters because there is not much to it. Follow them strictly and you will lose weight. As far as the tips in the back, try to follow as many as you can. They will help greatly.

First things first, familiarize yourself with the nutritional labels on food. If the food does not have a nutritional label and its not a veggie or fruit, do not eat it. Nutrition facts are required to be listed on the back of most foods. While you might think, "I know how to read nutrition labels." Stop right there and be sure to read the next section carefully. All of the information in this section should be taught in schools to children. I never learned how to read the nutrition labels correctly. I had to figure it out myself in my twenties. Too many people have no idea how to read the nutritional label in its' entirety. So, let's break it down.

Serving Size: This is most likely the most important portion of the nutrition label. Look at the serving size and see how much it consists of. Some things like: energy bars, drinks, small sized foods will be single-serving packages, meaning that the package only consists of ONE serving. But, occasionally you find something like a bag of chips that may have only 100 calories per serving and it will have TEN servings inside the bag. So if you eat this seemingly small bag of chips, you consume 1,000 calories. Serving sizes can be as small as one tablespoon, so pay attention. Be sure to see how big a tablespoon is when you are snacking on dip or some type of condiment.

Calories: Calories are important but not particularly in this lifestyle change because calories are just an overall sum of the fat, protein and carbs. In other words, the line that reads "Calories" is not too important because you will be adding up the calories by acknowledging the lines that read "Fat", "Carbohydrates", and "Protein". Each gram of fat is 9 calories. Each gram of protein or carbohydrate is 4 calories. For example if a food item has 10 grams of fat, no carbohydrates, and 2 grams of protein then it has 98 calories. Do not pay too much attention to the calories but rather what makes up the calories. After reading this section you should be able to know how many calories a food item has after looking at the fat, carbohydrate and protein content.

Total Fat: Fat is not always bad. It is grossly misunderstood. Fat can be a great source of energy. If you're like me, you splurge sometimes when it comes to fat. Whether its 1 bowl of ice cream or 1 candy bar the size of my small finger, the fat in that delicious treat is usually more than 30% of your daily-recommended fat intake. This is a HUGE deal. It doesn't seem like much, since when you glance a sweet treat it says "Only 200 calories!" But let's break fat down further, since not *all* fats are harmful to losing weight. The normal amount of calories a person should consume from fats is 30% of their daily calorie value. If you consume 2,000 calories a day then 600 of those calories can be fat. Some fats are good for you; they do not raise cholesterol or make you gain weight like bad fats do. Did you read that? Some fats are good for you and they do not raise cholesterol. First let us look at the bad fats; the fats you should avoid.

Saturated Fat: This is the most harmful fat for this lifestyle change. The difference between Unsaturated fat and Saturated fat is that Saturated fat is solid at room temperature and Unsaturated fat is liquid at room temperature. This means that if you know something is very fattening and it happens to be *solid*, it is most likely filled with saturated fat. Think about butter, it is solid and is basically just a glob of bad fat. Saturated fat not only makes you fat, but it can lead to cardiovascular disease. This is something to avoid at all costs but don't completely cut it out of your diet if you do not wish to.

Your food choices will be reconstructed by following this change and avoiding saturated fat will not be hard.

Unsaturated Fat: This fat is not always bad and it can be found in most energy filled food. It will be limited in the diet, but there is not much more you need to know about Unsaturated fat except it's still fat, just not as harmful to losing weight as many think. This will be discussed more in the Food section. Unsaturated fat is included in the Total Fat on the nutrition label: they will separate fats shown under Saturated fat, Trans Fat, Monounsaturated fat and Polyunsaturated fat.

Monounsaturated Fat: This fat, along with polyunsaturated fat, is considered one of the good fats and actually do exactly the opposite of Saturated and Trans fats. They lower risk for cardiovascular disease. These fats are your friends. Monounsaturated fats are found in a variety of food and oils that will be discussed in the food section. Remember, if you are looking for energy search for Monounsaturated fat.

Polyunsaturated Fat: These are incredibly beneficial. One polyunsaturated fat you've probably heard about is Omega-3's. These can be found in fatty fish and other various foods. Polyunsaturated fat will also be found in plant-based foods and oils. If you're wondering why you do not see Monounsaturated or Polyunsaturated fat on the back of your favorite food, it is because it does not contain any Polyunsaturated or Monounsaturated fat. These two fats will most likely be liquid at room temperature. Butter is a great example of a bad fat, it is solid at room temperature. Olive oil is a great example of a good fat, and it is liquid at room temperature. Ever wonder why nuts have a moisture-oily taste to them? That is because they are packed with healthy fats.

Cholesterol: This is a big one and can be more important depending on your age and prior eating habits. If you are very young you most likely do not have much to worry about cholesterol, but a steady high-cholesterol diet can lead to cardiovascular disease and high blood pressure. Most people don't know that your body produces cholesterol and you do not need ANY in your diet. Cholesterol is vital to your body because it helps produce hormones. But, as mentioned before, you do not need any in your diet since the body produces all you need to be healthy. It is recommended to get no more than 300mg of cholesterol each day and under 200mg if you are at risk for cardiovascular disease. If you have any more questions about cholesterol, please consult a doctor. I am not a doctor, therefore I can not give medical advice. Pay attention to cholesterol because just *one egg* is more then 60% of your daily value of cholesterol.

Some food items that may not be bad for you at all, considering they are low in sugar, low in fat – are packed with cholesterol! The chicken egg is a perfect example, as stated before just one egg can have more than 60% of your daily value of cholesterol. Most people eat 2 eggs when they have breakfast. That is 120% of your cholesterol for the day in one sitting: pay attention to your cholesterol intake.

Sodium: Don't worry too much about this one. It also can cause health problems in excess, much like cholesterol. If you have any kind of cardiovascular disease or any cardiovascular disease in your family then you need to pay more attention to your sodium intake. It is recommended that you get no more than 2,300mg of sodium everyday, which is one teaspoon of table salt. This is not a lifestyle change to lower cholesterol levels or blood pressure: please do not rely on it for such. If you have high blood pressure or cardiovascular disease please speak to a doctor before drastically changing your diet and lifestyle in accordance to this book.

Total Carbohydrate: Carbs are scary and there is a bunch of propaganda against them in the last decade but really, they are amazing for energy. They provide a sustainable long-lasting energy source. Don't get too excited, because there are two different types of carbs: simple and complex carbohydrates.

Simple carbohydrates are in simple terms the worst. They do not provide long lasting energy, and if you consume them they will temporarily spike glucose levels giving you a strong boost of energy for a short amount of time. This includes stuff like soda, honey and candy. This change in eating habits does not require you to completely stop eating these things, but it does limit your simple carb intake if you have a sweet tooth. Do NOT eat simple carbs before bed most importantly.

Complex carbohydrates are great and should be seen as your main source of energy. Complex carbs should make up roughly 50% or more of your daily calorie intake. These percentages are not too important, but it is helpful to know for some people. One interesting fact about carbs is that they actually use 23% of their consumed calories to store themselves if they are not used immediately. That means that carbs use a lot of their own calories to store themselves. If you do not use the carbs immediately and take a nap or hangout and watch TV, the carbs use a good amount of their own calories to store themselves. Whereas fat only uses 3% of its consumed calories to store itself. That is a huge difference. So, in other words, eat carbs over fat!

Fiber: Most Americans, I would assume, know what fiber is and what it does, but most people do not get enough. What you probably didn't know is, like every other nutritional component, it has two different types: soluble and insoluble. They are both good for you. Unlike fats, where you should intake monounsaturated and polyunsaturated more than trans or saturated fats, with fiber you can intake as much as you like of either kind! Fiber not only helps with the obvious reasons, clearing out your digestive system, but with lowering risk for disease.

Sugar: Ah, sugar. Sugar is usually everyone's favorite but it is not mine. My favorite is fat, good ol' saturated fat such as cheese enchiladas or a big double cheeseburger and fries. But most people have a serious sugar fix and a massive sweet tooth. We don't realize how much sugar is in everything. I am sure you know how much sugar is in a soda but did you know that a glass of orange juice (which has healthier, more natural sugar) has almost as much sugar as a glass of soda! This is something you need to be aware of and while you shouldn't focus on sugar, you should be conscience of the amount of sugar you are ingesting. It is easy to have a glass of orange juice or even a glass of milk before bed. Both of which has NO fat (if you're drinking skim milk), and this may sound like a delicious, nutritious snack but in fact it has massive amounts of sugar in it. Milk producers pack their products with sugar because they sacrifice fat. And they want their milk to taste the best. They do this on purpose. They trick their customer in to believing that the product is healthy because it has less fat, but in reality there is an insane amount of added sugar that is not natural to the milk. If you do not believe me, look it up. Adding sugar to drinks and food is a huge problem with food in America today.

Protein: This is a very important component much like carbs and fats. Most people think that if they ingest plenty of protein with little carbs or fat then they will be lean. I see so many people drinking protein shakes when they are trying to lose weight, but these people do not realize that protein is not even used until all carbs and fats have been used. Read that again: protein is not used until all carbs and fats have been used.

Chapter 2
FOOD

Now that you know how to add up calories by fat, protein, and carbs and how to distinguish between good carbs and bad carbs along with good fats and bad fats, the food section will seem only natural. In this section there will be lists of foods that are "good" and that you should focus on. This, of course, is based on a general understanding of very fatty foods and foods that do not provide a long-lasting source of energy.

Now it is time to get to the core of the actual weight loss. This next part will be what sets this lifestyle change apart from all the others and here are my secrets to losing weight quickly:

Breakfast – Eat a massive breakfast. This is going to be tricky at first but it will help you lose weight and fill full longer. There is a reason this is the first part of the Food Section because it is the most important part to this diet. If you do not follow these instructions you will not lose weight.

As you have probably heard, breakfast is the most important meal of the day and this is true. It is even truer for this specific dietary change. Breakfast is going to be your "cheat" meal. It will be your most fulfilling meal and also the only meal where you can go crazy. For people who do not normally eat breakfast or have a very small breakfast, this will be difficult. I use to not eat until midday and have a large lunch and an even larger dinner. This is going to reversed. Instead, you will be eating a huge breakfast, medium sized lunch and a very small, healthy dinner. Or maybe no dinner at all. Instead of eating 3 meals, you will be eating 2.

Huge breakfast? What does this mean? When I first started experimenting with this meal plan of a large breakfast, medium lunch and almost no dinner it was extremely hard for me to eat much in the morning. I simply was not hungry until later in the day. Here is the most fun part about this change: eat whatever you want for breakfast. I started out eating either eggs, hash browns and tortillas OR a big nutella filled crepe with bananas and strawberries; both of these meals accompanied by a tall glass of milk. If you want to have a bowl of ice cream along with a 3-egg veggie omelet and some pieces of whole wheat toast, DO IT. This may sound ridiculous but as you read on you will realize that by eating substantially less throughout the day you will compensate for these calories.

The main goal here is to begin accustoming your stomach to a large breakfast. At first, you may eat whatever you want. With ONE exception, you must eat something substantial so that means if you want to have a chocolate croissant be sure to eat a large bowl of healthy yogurt with granola and fruit. Eat something that is packed with long-lasting carbs, fats and protein along side of your treat. Be careful with yogurt, it is a great thing to eat but be sure to pick a healthy one. Look at the back, notice how much sugar it contains. Do not look for the yogurt that says "No Fat", instead look for the yogurt that has little sugar and some fat. Add your own sugar such as honey, fruit, or granola. Breakfast should be the meal you feel most full after. Eventually your body will wake up starving and breakfast will become your favorite meal of the day.

Lunch – This meal is going to be easy because while you can't eat *whatever* you want, like you could with breakfast, you do not have to starve yourself. Remember how calories work, when you go to the grocery store do not buy things that are ridiculously packed with bad fats or simple carbs unless you plan to eat it for breakfast along side other energy packed food.

Lunch should be something like a sandwich or pasta (try to use whole wheat pasta and bread always). This meal is at your discretion. You should be able to make an educated decision as to what to eat. One helpful tip: cut out the cheese. If you have to eat cheese, look for cheese that is either very thin and has less than 15% of your daily fat value. This will most likely be labeled reduced fat, and it is hard to find. Most cheeses have 30% of your daily fat value PER a slice or every 1/4th cup if its shredded: This is insanity!

What do you put on your sandwich? What should you put in your pasta? This, again, you should be able to answer since you now know how to read nutritional information. Later, there will be a comprehensive list of food you should start to love and try to stick to regarding meats and proteins. It will be food that is low in fat and is a complete protein. A complete protein means that it contains the 9 essential amino acids that every human needs to survive. This is why if you speak to any veteran vegetarian they are well versed in complete proteins because when you only eat vegetables it is hard to get the essential amino acids. Your sandwich could be turkey, chicken or some other lean meat. Your pasta could have the same meats with a light sauce. A peanut butter and jelly sandwich is also a good alternative. Peanut butter and whole wheat bread combine to make a complete protein. It is important that you make sure any kind of grain or pasta is whole grain. You want those complex carbs, not simple carbs!

This diet is all about meal distribution and relative dieting. Relative dieting means that you're not trying to cut out all the calories in your day, you are just trying to eat less daily than you did the year before. If you are the type of person that has roughly 2,500 calories a day and you have been eating that way for over 5 years, than you will have great success eating 2,000 healthier calories every day.

When I was told that in order to lose weight that I needed a 500 calorie deficit everyday (meaning that I must burn more calories than I eat) I was stunned. Not only was this crazy because I was unhealthy and never exercised, but it showed me that the nutritionist I was speaking to had no idea what he was talking about. In order for someone who is already overweight and unhealthy to lose weight, all they need to do is eat less than they did the day before and get some type of easy, mild exercise. After lunch comes…

Dinner – This is usually a person's largest meal. You miss breakfast, have a compensating lunch, then typically by the time it gets to the evening, you are starving. Following this booklet, you will not be starving by the time you get to dinner. Another key to this diet, along with a massive breakfast and understanding nutritional information, is <u>cutting out dinner</u>.

Cutting out dinner. This might sound frightening but trust me it's not that bad. I do not mean eat nothing for dinner, I just mean that you should keep it very small and healthy. Skip it completely when you can. Go to bed earlier. The earlier you go to bed, the sooner you will wake up for your favorite meal: breakfast! This will allow your body to burn off those extra calories while you sleep and it will also make your stomach look forward to your breakfast. On top of that, more sleep will help your body in countless ways. At first, this may be very difficult because you will find that your body is use to having a large dinner. But I promise once you cut out dinner for a few days you will immediately see results in your weight loss. Dinner from now on can be something like a salad, a small sandwich, a serving of lean meat, or as many servings of vegetables as you like. I tend to have half a peanut butter and jelly sandwich. While this may sound like something a small bird would eat, you will be surprised at how much you look forward to a half of a sandwich once you have cut yourself off from eating multiple servings at dinner.

Don't go to bed with a rumbling, starved stomach because this will not allow you to sleep well. Try not to have sugar *right* before bed, this includes fruits, but something like a piece of whole grain toast with half a tablespoon of peanut butter or half an avocado with salt and lemon will keep you from getting bad sleep.

Once you have cut your dinner down, try to eat less and less until you are able to still have energy from breakfast and lunch. Dinner should become something like a bowl of veggies or a salad.

This part of the dietary change will be very difficult for most people, but it is one of the most important parts. Once you have cut down your dinner substantially, you will see results immediately.

In the next part I will have a long list of foods that you should focus on but through understanding how calories work you should be able to make your own list of favorite, healthy foods. This is not a strict list and you are allowed to veer from it. It helps a lot of people to be able to see a list so I will include one. The idea is to eat healthier daily than you did the year before. If you have been eating cheese pizza and garlic knots every Thursday for the past year then you will try to eat a veggie pizza with light cheese on Thursdays. The whole point is trying to reduce portions and redistribute your calories.

PROTEIN

BEEF
Lean cuts, such as:
Eye of Round
Ground beef: Lean
Pastrami, lean
Sirloin Steak
Tenderloin
Top Loin
Top Round

POULTRY
Chicken
Cornish hen
Turkey bacon
Turkey sausage

Turkey and chicken breast

SEAFOOD
All types of fish and shellfish are good

PORK
Boiled ham
Canadian bacon
Loin
Tenderloin

VEAL
Chop Cutlet, leg
Top round

LAMB
Center Cut
Chop
Loin

LUNCHMEAT
Fat-free or low-fat - Look around; you will find some with less fat, that does not look terrible and it will have 30-50% less fat than the contemporaries.

MEAT SUBSTITUTES (SOY BASED)
Look for things with low fat but most of the time this is the best option. Soy substitutes do not taste good to some people, but it is something everyone should try. If you like it, you'll have a great time losing weight.

As for <u>CARBOHYDRATES and FAT</u>, these are at your discretion and remember how to get healthy carbs and fats. Whole grain pasta, types of granolas, and nuts are all fine as long as you pay attention how much you are ingesting. Find a great granola that you can put in yogurt or eat with some soy milk, almond milk or regular milk. It should have a low amount of sugar and high amount of fiber. When you are at the grocery store, pick up a few different brands and compare. It will be amazing how self-efficient you feel finding the best one.

Also, remember that fruits and vegetables will have carbohydrates and fats. This should be your main source for simple carbs. Try to have a breakfast or lunch packed with fruits or vegetables. It is important you get both vegetables and fruits, but breakfast is your time to cheat. You can put butter or chocolate on them. Do not have it the other way around: where you have ice cream, fruit, and chocolate sauce for dessert after dinner.

Look for vegetables, fruits, and nuts that have polyunsaturated fat and monounsaturated fat. These will provide great energy throughout the day. These will surprise you because most of them taste good and fill you up.

If you have a favorite or a couple favorite fruit/vegetables start to focus on these heavily. For example, if you like bananas then start having a couple bananas everyday. I know it is sometimes hard to remember to eat fruit or vegetables but you must have plenty of them around, always fresh and visible, in order to start eating them.

Try to eat 1-3 servings of fruit and/or vegetable for your first meal. It will provide a lot of natural sugars that will wake up your body as well as your mind.

Chapter 3
MOVE

This is the shortest part of the booklet. It is not meant to scare you. The most important parts to this lifestyle change are the reformation of your concept on food, and changing your biggest meal to breakfast while cutting out dinner. In order to lose weight, remember 75% of it depends on your eating habits and only 25% of the weight loss depends on exercising.

But working out cannot be neglected. Everything is relative. For instance, if you already work out 2-3 times a week for roughly an hour then all this calls for is expanding your cardio.

If you do not work out at all and you do not want to work out, then you should start doing one of the best fat-burning exercises known to man: walking. Walking a couple miles, in a sense, burns more fat than running a mile. Low intensity cardio burns more fat, but not as many calories as high intensity cardio like running. This does not mean that you are burning more calories walking for 20 minutes than a marathon runner, but it does mean that walking is a great way to lose a LOT of weight. Spending 10 minutes running a mile only burns around 100 calories. You should be briskly walking for 30 minutes or more and burning hundreds of calories. The longer you can walk, the better.

Walk if you do not do anything else. Try to do this everyday. It will not only make you feel good being outside, but it will increase your motivation since you can feel the fat burning off. There is something empowering about getting outside and moving. The sun is also a big factor in this lifestyle change because it provides us with vitamins that are otherwise hard to get into the body. Physical activity has great benefits for the body but also for the mind.

Working out is great, and by working out I mean lifting weights or playing sports, which are kinds of higher intensity cardio. These are important, but in order to lose weight try to lengthen your workouts. It does not mean that you need to start lifting twice as much weight, or that your work out has to be twice as long. It means that you should add time to your workout by taking a brisk walk or jog, on top of your normal muscle building exercises. Focus on the fat to sculpt and lose weight. Focus on muscle to build.

Chapter 4
TIPS

1) Water – Drink it. If you feel hungry and you know you should not eat, drink a full glass of water. It will temporary curve your appetite and it helps every vital organ in your body run properly. Secondly, cold water is the <u>only</u> negative calorie drink. The body burns calories to warm the cold water once you ingest it. Remember this and take it to heart. I read that the body burns up to 6.8 calories per 8oz glass of ice water. That means that if you drank 10 glasses of cold ice water everyday, you would be burning 68 calories doing absolutely nothing. It may not sound like a lot but it is! Running one mile burns roughly 100 calories.

2) Eat a massive breakfast – I cannot stress this enough. Fill yourself once a day. You should only feel full one time during the day and that is after breakfast.

3) Bread Veggies – If you hate vegetables like I do then you are wondering how you are going to get your fiber and vegetables for the day. Try breading vegetables. Buy breadcrumbs in the store and use a vegetable like eggplant, zucchini, cauliflower, etc. All you need to do it slice the vegetable, dip it in egg then dip it in breadcrumbs, and finally put it in a pan on the stove with a bit of healthy oil such as corn oil. Cook each side for 3-4 minutes over a medium-low flame. It is a delicious alternative to steamed vegetables.

4) Juicing – Look into juicing vegetables or find a juice bar near by. It is a great way to take down a pound of vegetables without actually having to eat them. There are tons of benefits to juicing vegetables. Start juicing now.

5) Reduced Fat or Reduced Sugar – Almost every food you buy has a reduced fat or reduced sugar option. These will greatly cut down your unhealthy calorie intake. Whenever you buy anything at the grocery store, look for the reduced fat or reduced sugar item. Never buy butter again unless it is made with oil or some healthier substitute. The only thing you need to be careful of is added sugar when you see something that is Reduced Fat. As I mentioned earlier in the book, a lot of yogurts do this. They might say "No Fat" but when compared to a yogurt that does have fat, the "No Fat" yogurt has exponentially more sugar. It is ok to have a little natural fat rather than having something pumped with added sugar.

6) Boxes of Pasta – These are awesome meals. They can be found in all kinds of different varieties from fettuccine alfredo to mac and cheese to garlic and olive oil vermicelli. But wait, when you look at the back of the box some of these pastas have, in one serving, 20-60% of your daily fat?! Here is the secret. Most of these boxes of pasta when you prepare them say to add 2-3 tablespoons of butter. Two to three tablespoons of butter! That is a ton of butter and unhealthy fat. I tried something crazy when I found these pastas, I made it without the butter and it tasted delicious. There is only one problem with these pastas and that is since they are not whole grain. They do not keep you full for long. Add some breaded veggies to them or lean meat, and you will be very full after this meal.

7) Popcorn – The best snack for weight loss. Get popcorn with light butter or no butter. Examine the nutritional information on the back. Popcorn has less calories when it is popped then when it is not popped. The amount of popcorn in one bag is gigantic, if a bag of popcorn does not fill you up for a snack then nothing will. It has healthy fats and plenty of fiber. Popcorn gets a bad wrap because most people thing about the popcorn you get at the movies, which is covered in liquid butter. In reality though, popcorn popped in the microwave at home does not have nearly as many calories. Just look at the back of a popcorn box and read the nutritional label: you'll notice it has healthy fats and almost no bad calories.

8) Suck it in – This is an old trick. From now on your should try to suck in your stomach only 1 centimeter. That is half the length of a penny. Why? Because it will make you conscience of your stomach muscles and by doing this it will strengthen your core. It won't give you abs or be the equivalent of a workout. All this is going to do is tighten up your core slowly. You are doing this for yourself, not for others. You will be able to feel it aching after trying to do it all day. Try to suck in your stomach whenever you remember, it will help.

9) Fruit – This is something most people don't focus on. They get one or two fruits and go on their way to the other aisles at the grocery store. What you probably have not noticed is how expensive everything is in the grocery store when compared to fruit. Fruit is incredibly inexpensive. You can spend a few dollars on pounds of fruit. Do not skip the fruit section because you do not want to waste money on something that will go bad in less than a week. Pile up on fruit. Next step: make it visible. I constantly stick fruit in the drawers in the refrigerator. That is the worst place for fruit. Why did the people who made refrigerators make it so the fruit is basically hidden below all the other stuff? If you walk in to the kitchen and the first thing you see is fruit then you are more likely to eat it. Keep fruit in the front of a shelf in the refrigerator or in a bowl on the kitchen counter. Put a ton of fruit right in front of your face, that way if you do not eat it immediately at least it will make you feel guilty about wasting it. It works; trust me.

10) Asian Food – I'm a food lover. I see what is on the food network at least once a day. I particularly enjoy the shows where a fat guy goes to a city and gobbles up local eateries. Something I noticed is no matter where this guy ventures, the ingredients to the pancakes, burgers, pizzas, or whatever he is eating on that particular day usually include a huge amount of butter, cheese, or cream. Not only do they use butter or cheese on the completed product but they usually use some type of fat in the initial ingredients. Except for when he goes to a place that has Asian cuisine. This would be some place like Thai, Japanese, Vietnamese, or even Chinese. At these restaurants, they typically do not even have butter in the kitchen. They use oils, sauces, and spices instead. Another thing I noticed while watching these shows is that typically the chef in the Asian restaurants are half the size of the chefs in the other restaurants. Now, do not start thinking you can eat orange chicken and fried rice every night because some of these dishes have been incredibly Americanized. Go for tofu Pad Thai or a bowl of Vietnamese seafood Pho. Both of these can be incredibly tasty. With Pad Thai, there is an amazing peanut sauce on the noodles and vegetables. With Pho, you can eat it plain, or put sweet plum sauce and sriracha on it. These sauces may have fat (from peanuts) or sugar (from plums), but that is much healthier than eating something that has little to no nutritional value and a huge amount of saturated fat.

11) The Internet – We have been given a great tool and that is the internet. If you do not know if a food is healthy or if you want to know which food is healthier when you are comparing: go to the internet. Every time I have a question like, "Is a regular potato or a sweet potato better for you?" I type it into my browser. It seems like 99.9% of my questions have already been asked and answered then fact checked by the masses. If you are unsure about something, ask. If you find anything that this book has proclaimed to be unbelievable, look it up on the internet. Clinical studies, nutritionists, doctors, personal trainers, and people with real life experience are all readily available on the internet.

Chapter 5
STORIES

Story About Fruit

One day I was sitting in a small lecture and everyone started to discuss diets. I kept my mouth shut because I wanted to hear what they had to say. One particularly plump girl started to go on about how certain fruits were bad for you. Yes, fruits that are bad for you. I couldn't believe my ears. She went on to say that apples were in fact awful for losing weight because they make you hungry. She claimed that she did not eat apples because they made you hungrier. If she is avoiding a fruit then what is her alternative? A piece of pizza, a hamburger? At least a piece of pizza or a hamburger would not make her hungrier, like an apple would. That was her reasoning.

Story About Fat

A friend of mine is a chef. He has been a chef for years. He cooks for people like you and me behind the doors of restaurants' kitchens. He is a great cook regardless of this story. We began to speak about a tomato soup that he was taught how to prepare. I began to ask him if it was healthy: did it have butter? did it use real tomatoes? Assuring me it had no butter, he informed me that it was grossly unhealthy because it was fattening. The soup had olive oil in it, instead of butter. I was appalled that someone in this position did not know the difference between healthy fats and unhealthy fats. He went on to claim that no matter what kind of fat it was, it still raised your cholesterol. Wrong.

You've Heard This Before

It is too often when I am contemplating what to eat with a friend I hear the same thing. Sometimes they will know we are trying to eat healthy, sometimes they will not. I might say something like "Oh, the Caesar salad sounds good." And they will say, "That is not good for you, it has so much Parmesan cheese and dressing!" That may be true. But, if I do not eat this salad what am I going to eat instead? You have to make sure you are going for the healthiest option; it does not have to be perfection. Sure, a burger with lecture, tomato, onions, and pickles may be unhealthy, but it is healthier than the double bacon burger with fries. Many people will try to say something is unhealthy because of an ingredient. What they do not realize is that without that ingredient such as dressing, you may neglect certain food groups that your body needs to stay healthy.

Final Note: Remember this text does not speak about the dangers of processed foods, sugar, and sodium extensively. If you have questions about these things, seek a professional's help. Good luck!

www.ingramcontent.com/pod-product-compliance
Lightning Source LLC
Chambersburg PA
CBHW030550290526
45786CB00004B/1953